AF730755

THE HUMAN DIET REBOOT

What Are Picky Eaters Trying to Tell Us

GREGORY STYPKO

Copyright © 2019 Gregory Stypko
All Rights Reserved.
ISBN:
ISBN-13: 978-0-578-50249-6

To Picky Eaters

Have you tried turning it off and on again?
— **The IT Crowd**

TABLE OF CONTENTS

Introduction

Why do we need to reboot our diet? Simply put, the fundamentals of our eating habits are seriously flawed. They are based on agrarian eating traditions rather than our nomadic Stone Age eating practices. Yet we use this faulty base to define our modern diets, and we know how those are working for us. Consuming different fat, carbohydrate and protein ratios, excluding certain foods, and adding extra vitamins, superfoods and supplements can't fix our diet. We must go all the way back to how our eating patterns evolved and start there. We must reboot our diet to the natural eating pattern of our Stone Age ancestors.

Contrary to prevailing opinions, the original human diet is identifiable. It stands apart from other regimens because besides offering general guidance on what to eat, it defines how we should do it. Our natural pattern of food ingestion is more important than what is on the menu because it makes us better tolerate our meals. The lessened dependence on specific foods used to be hugely advantageous, as it allowed our ancestors all around the globe to thrive on a wide range of local foods. However, we, in search of a perfect diet, obsess mostly over food choice and macronutrient ratios, not noticing that we are consuming them the wrong way. The result is a head-spinning variety of regimens that vary marginally in their health benefits. In certain circumstances, and for some people, one regimen seems better than another. We falsely attribute those benefits to the inherent qualities of the diets themselves, but we don't consider that change itself could be helping our digestion, regardless of the diets we switch between. The menu-change-benefits-digestion concept agrees nicely with the philosophy of our natural regimen.

Let me tell you a little about my dietary experiences. In my search for a better diet, I tried a few regimens, including low-carbohydrate, paleo and keto diets. I felt slightly better each time after the switch, but the difference wasn't overwhelming, and I still couldn't shed the extra pounds. The change to the natural diet, while harder, was incomparable when it came to the results. In the way I look and feel, compared to other diets I tried, our prototypical regimen is in a different league. Once I experienced the steadiness of mood throughout the day, the lack of mental fog, headaches and digestive symptoms, I knew that I had found my natural diet. I also see a difference when I look in the mirror. My skin is more even, not too dry and not too oily, my dark spots have faded, and other cosmetic dermatological problems—that I was told by my doctor to just live with—are barely noticeable. Even my sweat smells different. That is, it doesn't smell at all. Strangely enough, as I appreciated all aspects of my physiological transformation, the neutrality of my sweat finally convinced me I am functioning on my natural diet.

This book is my second about our natural diet. The previous one, *The Food Bondage: Making a Case for the Human Diet*, advocates bringing back the structure of our natural diet to counteract the obesity epidemic. *The Food Bondage*, as its title suggests, focuses on current nutritional dysfunction, and delves deeply into the link between our food dependency and our unnatural food consumption model.

The Human Diet Reboot is focused more on the diet itself, transitioning to it and functioning on it in our current circumstances. In this book, I will discuss different aspects of our natural diet. The first job of this book is to convince you that what I propose is, in fact, the original human diet. I will present you with a chain of logic that leads to that conclusion. Then I will describe my dietary struggles, research, and experimentation, which eventually directed me toward our natural diet. Finally, I will show you the tactics that one may use when switching to our natural diet—and living with it. This book necessarily overlaps with the previous one. However, in the year since I comprehended our natural nutrition, I developed further arguments to substantiate it. One of them is the resistance which our kids put up when we train them to eat three daily meals. Although I mentioned it in the previous book, I realized since then this behavior is more significant than I had initially thought. Now I am convinced that our kids—the picky eaters—should be our heroes. Those tiny tots who spit their food out and torment us with their refusal to eat by the clock are telling us how much we have strayed from our natural eating habits.

Having had more time to reflect on the different aspects of the diet and to experience it for another year, I am not only convinced of the superiority of our natural dietary framework but also of the inevitability of its eventual acceptance as the nutritional standard.

CHAPTER ONE

Dietary Landscape

The variety of diets out there is astounding. There are so many that they have rankings. *U.S. News & World Report*, for example, allows readers to rank them by goal (weight loss, diabetes, heart-healthy, etc.), type (balanced, high-protein, low-calorie, low-carbohydrate, etc.) and preference (alcohol allowed, easy to follow, gluten-free, exercise recommended, etc.).

Our idea of correct nutrition is a big, confusing jumble of ideas pointing in different directions. I used to be a keen follower of dietary discourse. I was fascinated by many qualified people coming to radically different conclusions about nutrition. When presenting their views, the experts typically delve deeply into the details of our digestion and metabolism to substantiate their claims. To support their diets, they present wellness evaluations of people who have switched to their favored regimen. The tests apparently confirm subjects' health improvement. It's all quite impressive, but it leads nowhere. New, promising diets pop up and fade away while our eating recommendations stay the same.

Our nutritional disarray is triggered by the fact that our officially recommended diet doesn't work for many people. This has spurred the quest for a better alternative. However, the human body is extremely complex. Plus, our approach seems to be the head-on analysis of the details of the body's life processes. Due to gaps in our understanding of nutrition, the experts have come to divergent conclusions based on their incomplete knowledge of various parts of the gigantic nutritional puzzle. It's time to change our perspective. How difficult was the problem of nutrition for early humans?

Unlike us, they were not overthinking their diet, as they had little choice. Our roving forebears' life circumstances imposed a specific eating pattern. Therefore, looking closely at their environment, we can indirectly discover their dining behaviors. That dietary structure is key to understanding our optimal nutrition.

In contrast to the nomadic circumstances of enforced food consumption, early farmers had a choice in how to eat their food stocks. Based on that, they invented a convenient and comforting way of consuming food we are, unfortunately, following today.

Our modern diet results from our civilizational progress. Our ancestors' goal was to feed more people in a predictable manner. They farmed to make themselves less dependent on nature. Who wants to travel for miles, change hunting grounds and foraging areas, only to face the same unpredictability of nature in every new region and with every changing season? From gorging themselves in the summer when exploiting bountiful areas, to having barely adequate meals in spring and fall, to almost starving in the mostly barren winter, the life of the Stone Age nomads was precarious.

The roving lifestyle was harsh and couldn't consistently feed very many people. Our ancestors wanted stability and efficiency in their food supply, and that was achieved when our forebears cultivated their crops and engaged in animal husbandry. Naturally, having food on-hand almost always, as their nomadic predecessors had not, our farmer forefathers ate differently. The nomads had to procure their meals piecemeal, and when they did, they would eat them promptly. The farmers, on the other hand, prepared their food stocks for the year to eat them whenever was convenient.

Unfortunately, our farming ancestors outsmarted themselves. They broke the natural human eating pattern. They thought that since they didn't have to procure their meals daily, they could eat early, and instead of having to work on an empty stomach, they could eat beforehand. Our custom of three daily meals probably evolved gradually. As more food was available and more people could afford eating more frequently, the number of meals finally settled on three. That number seems to make sense, as it keeps us feeling relatively full between meals, but how healthy is it?

CHAPTER TWO

Root of Dietary Evil

We are amidst an unprecedented nutrition-related health crisis. Millions of us get sick because we overeat. We realize the consequences of overeating and the U.S. Department of Agriculture tells us precisely what to do to prevent it. So, why don't we heed that advice? Why do we consistently and massively overeat?

Here is a possible explanation. Our environment and eating instincts shape our eating behavior. We—modern people—inherited our eating instincts from our nomadic ancestors. For Stone Age nomads, calorie-dense foods were exceptional. Therefore, they developed the instinct to pack in those calorie bombs to survive the inevitably ensuing leaner times. This instinct is not unique to humans. It is the same drive that makes the bears and other mammals build fat reserves for the winter. For our nomadic ancestors, the conditions of food availability were such that occasional calorie-bomb's overconsumption was critical to their survival.

For us—modern humans—the food consumption environment is entirely different. We have plenty of highly-caloric foods that are available all year-round. And they are heavily advertised, cheap and available on nearly every corner. However, our instinct to overeat is the same as our, genetically, almost identical nomadic ancestors.

It looks like this powerful survival drive utterly defeats, for most of us, our conscious attempts to reign it in. How should we view, in that context, our dietary advice?

We are advised to eat mostly starchy meals three times daily, with snacking between if necessary. We are being encouraged to eat regularly throughout the day while in the same breath, we are being told to restrain ourselves by choosing lower-calorie foods and limit our caloric intake. Eating steadily starch-based meals makes it very difficult to fight the overeating instinct. What if our natural regimen made it much easier to overcome our overeating drive?

I contend that our currently recommended way of food consumption is suboptimal, and that is an understatement. I consider our official dietary advice as pointing us toward the opposite of the natural human diet. Why? Because it differs so significantly from our natural eating regimen. However, most health professionals would consider the natural nomadic regimen unhealthy. Is it?

Let's consider three meals daily. How was it possible before the farming revolution? It wasn't; our nomadic ancestors couldn't have eaten regular, frequent meals. Therefore, our current diet is unnatural because, at its core, is the assumption of constant food availability. If, from the modern diet perspective, the notions of skipping meals and fasting are unhealthy, what can we say about our modern diet from the nomadic diet perspective?

Which dietary structure is healthier for humans—the natural diet to which they had adapted through evolution or the artificial one that they've switched to because of the steady food supply?

To realize how unnatural our diet is, let's start with our childhood. We train our children to eat regular meals—and they resist. If you are a parent or have watched one feeding their infant child, you'll know what I mean. In time, children adjust to the scheduled eating pattern. However, that trained behavior goes against our natural adaptation.

It's not surprising that, after decades of three meals daily, our bodies adjust to that pattern—both physically and mentally. Our GI tract, metabolic system and brain accommodate constant digestion; it feels normal. Therefore, it's to be expected that when we attempt to skip a meal, we react poorly. We get distracted, get a headache or feel weak. The older we get, the more we become reliant on the meal regularity.

Is it possible to go back to our natural diet in today's reality? Yes, it is. However, it requires unlearning the dietary rules which we've been trained to follow. As to the health implications of the diet switch, the honest answer is nobody knows. Sure, there are confirmed health benefits of the keto diet and fasting, but those were not subject to extensive dietary studies yet, and it doesn't look like they will be anytime soon. So, effectively, we have a *Catch-22* situation here. We can't recommend alternative eating behaviors because they were not tested on large populations, and finding a large population following them is impossible because they are not officially recommended.

However, consider both diets and decide which one makes more sense. For our natural diet speaks our evolutionary adaptation. For the recommended regimen a millennia-old agrarian eating tradition. We must eat in a specific way to live optimally healthy lives. Emulating eating habits that our Paleolithic ancestors followed for over two million years is more important than we are led to believe. Many people already experiment with and recommend some of the aspects of our natural diet.

The proponents of fasting, OMAD and keto value them as effective means of health improvement. However, no one places those individual dietary behaviors in a broader context. Therefore, we can't see the whole picture of our natural eating framework and don't understand how and why its individual components come together. In the subsequent chapters, I will do that and also bring to your attention unpublicized details of our ancestral diet that are critically important.

Before I continue, let's examine different meanings of the word diet. One of them stands for all aspects of food consumption—both the foods and the way we consume them. The other is just the foods.

I will use the word diet or regimen to mean all aspects of food consumption. I will apply the word menu to food selection, and the words structure, framework or pattern will refer to the way we consume foods. That is the eating frequency and macronutrients ratios of meals.

The U.S. Department of Agriculture nutritional guidelines recommend a diet. Most of us assume this advice is based on scientific studies—and here is a curious thing; it is and it isn't. The framework of the diet isn't as it's derived from our agrarian eating tradition. However, based on that structure, the experts evaluate different food combinations and calorie intakes and recommend to us what they consider the best variant.

I have a problem with accepting the framework of the diet unquestioningly and starting evaluation from the details of its implementation. In the nutritional guidelines, there is a reference to dietary recommendations as science-based nutrition. I am not quite sure of how much that statement reflects reality. However, as I am not capable of a thorough scientific evaluation of my proposed natural diet, I am satisfied describing it as logic-based nutrition.

It's indisputable that our traditional three-meals-daily starch-based diet is not our natural one as it's created around our staple crops. Also, it's certain that we are genetically adapted to a nomadic diet. What does it mean in practice? That our GI tract and the metabolic system evolved to work optimally with a specific ingestion frequency and meals macronutrient profile.

Our eating adaptation comes from millions of years of our Stone Age ancestors living a nomadic lifestyle. Contrary to many of today's opinions that portray their lives as an idyllic, almost carefree existence, the survival in the wild couldn't have been easy. Some of our idealized thinking about our Stone Age ancestors may stem from observing our contemporary quasi-nomads. Most of the indigenous people today we think of as nomads are semi-nomads. Therefore, their eating habits are halfway between our traditional and a nomadic way of food consumption. Their dietary behavior doesn't represent accurately that of the actual Stone Age roving humans.

CHAPTER THREE

We Are Nomads

That we, on average, live much longer than our nomadic forefathers doesn't mean that much. It doesn't reflect the robustness of our shared physique. We must realize that our roving forbears used to live in much harsher circumstances. Almost everything related to their external conditions was working against them. Between their infant mortality, miles they had to walk or run, the injuries and infections they sustained, uneven food quality, toxins, insect bites, exposure to elements including frostbite and sunburn, vitamin deficiencies, severe starvation and dehydration, many factors jeopardized their survival and accelerated their aging. Also, their coddled childhood was most likely much shorter than today's kids. In that context, when we reflect on our lives today, we see how overbuilt our bodies are for our current lives. Our bodies evolved to withstand harsh conditions for many years. That also included a not always salubrious dietary reality.

Predictably, the lives of our nomadic ancestors revolved around food, as our lives do, but in a different way. Instead of mostly thinking about what to select for the next meal, they had a much harder time making it happen. That next meal wasn't a given, and its content depended on the time of the year, a specific area they were in and luck. Therefore, their digestive system was accustomed to fasts of different durations, as well as undereating and overeating. The word accustomed isn't strong enough here. Because the conditions in which they lived lasted for millions of years, their GI tracts, metabolism and the rest of their bodies adjusted themselves to work optimally under those variable conditions. Those conditions of unsteady availability and quality of sustenance are similar for all wild animals. It’s a consequence of being, to a large degree, at the mercy of nature.

Due to our speedy civilizational progress since the end of the Stone Age, it's hard to grasp that this period of our ancestors having at their disposal only simple tools and weapons is responsible for our development as humans. It is startling to think that Stone Age people had the same intellectual capacity as we do for learning, memorizing, thinking abstractly and the capability to have rich emotional lives as we do. Our nurturing makes us modern people but, deep down, our genetics still define us as nomads. Therefore, we can't change what's best for our bodies. We can use our bodies differently, and they will adapt to a certain degree, but that won't mean they will work optimally under the new conditions.

There is a broad range of suboptimal behaviors that our bodies will accommodate, we know that. Many of us smoke and drink and our organs, for many decades, can cope with the incoming toxins. It's easy to imagine how health-promoting less abusive behaviors are. Between our robust organs and malleable brains, we can accommodate for long periods those less-than-optimal circumstances. Isn't it any wonder that we can tolerate unnatural diets?

One way of illustrating optimal and suboptimal conditions is to imagine a short line with a point in the middle. The point is where our organ works optimally, like our heart beating at 100 beats per minute. To the left and to the right our heart beats slower and faster. Let's say the left end of the line is marked 60 bpm. The right end of the line would be 200 bpm. Most of the time, we would like to stay close to that middle 100 bpm mark. However, occasionally our heart would beat slower or faster. However, staying for a long time close to the extremes wouldn't be optimal, perhaps even dangerous.

Now imagine our GI tract. The point in the middle is marked one. That is the typical nomadic frequency of the meals. The point on the left is marked zero, that is no meal. The point to the right is three, that is three meals daily. Now imagine that we stay on mark three for our whole lives. What are the possible consequences for our digestive system?

Imagine our mouth, esophagus, stomach, small intestine, liver, gallbladder, and pancreas at rest for near twenty hours on mark one. Now, imagine the upper digestive system being at rest for less than twelve hours—mostly when we sleep. Otherwise, the upper GI tract is working; starting from breakfast, virtually constantly if counting our beverages and snacks.

Now add to that picture our ancestors fasting for a day or few. Those complete shutdowns of our digestion are programmed into the optimal operation of our GI tract. From the sporadic mode of operation optimal for our species, we've moved it to the continual and that makes a huge difference.

I will show in later chapters the extent to which our traditional dietary structure differs from the nomadic one. I am sure that nutrition experts know of a discrepancy but, apparently, in their opinion, the difference is not that significant. Still it would seem prudent to consider our nomadic diet as worthy of emulation. So, why don't our dietary authorities nomadize our eating recommendations? The usual rationale given is that our living circumstances changed so much that it's impossible to recreate the nomadic diet exactly. Here is where the discussion gets interesting.

Remember that we use the word diet to mean different concepts—the menu and the whole aspect of food consumption, which is both the how and what we eat.

When considering our inability to recreate the pre-agrarian diet, most people have in mind the forgotten nomadic foods, and those are indeed almost impossible to identify. However, as I will show later in the book, we can determine the other, an arguably more important aspect of the pre-agrarian diet—the eating pattern. As to the foods, what if knowing them is not that important? I postulate that the core of our menu and the nomadic food selection are equivalent. Our nomadic ancestors could do just fine on the bulk of today's food products. That makes sense if we assume that they and we are genetically almost identical. Some over-processed foods would harm them just as they hurt us. However, our veggies, fruit, nuts, eggs, meat, fish and even grain would be suitable for them.

Disregarding sugar and over-processed starches and fats, most of our standard meals, like homecooked dinners, are processed to roughly the same degree as those of our nomadic ancestors'. That is because our teeth and digestive systems are virtually the same. If we can consume them and stay reasonably healthy when we don't overeat, so could they. I contend that we would do much better if we consumed those same foods the nomadic way and, as importantly, it would make it easier to limit our calorie intake when eating like nomads. To sum it up, modern foods should not prevent us from significantly benefiting from the nomadic diet structure. Contrary to many popular opinions, we should be emulating how they were eating not what they were eating.

I have read many opinions on how bad today's foods are compared to those of our nomadic predecessors. That opinion is not about junk food but the foods we consider healthy. I don't agree with that assessment. I think that we idealize our pre-agrarian living circumstances and food processing skills of our nomadic ancestors. Most of today's healthy meals are better for us than what our roving ancestors would typically eat. Because of their farming origin, modern plant foods may contain smaller amounts of minerals and vitamins than their wild equivalents. The same somewhat lower quality standard applies to the meat of our farmed-raised animals, but our modern foods are also cleaner, have consistent nutritional quality and most likely contain fewer natural toxins. As for the content of vitamins and minerals, our veggies fruit and meats provide more than enough. That many of us take extra vitamins and minerals just in case is unfortunate because, for many, it's how they compensate for bad dietary choices.

Remember that our nomadic forebears didn't have steady access to high-quality foods. Therefore, in a pinch, they had to eat lower quality meals consisting of a little too fibrous, microbially contaminated or even somewhat toxic nourishments. We seem to forget that nature didn't create veggies, fruit, and meats already suitable for our digestion—we did. Who do you think, mostly, could do a better job adapting wild flora and fauna for human consumption? The Stone Age humans or us modern people?

So, if our foods are not the problem, what is? As mentioned, it's the way we eat our meals. We should change our eating pattern. We shouldn't be eating according to our frequent schedule with roughly the same fat/carbohydrate/protein content all year-round. That eating pattern, although simplistically logical and comforting, is unnatural. It reflects our distorted-through-constant-food-availability-thinking about healthy nutrition. It's unlike the way our nomadic ancestors used to feed themselves. Our eating pattern is not only suboptimal regarding our digestive and metabolic systems, but also highly conducive to overeating. By adopting the eating habits of the Stone Age nomads, we could have the best of both diets—our modern, consistent-quality foods and consume them the optimal way of our nomadic ancestors.

CHAPTER FOUR

Hunger Confusion

Different cravings motivate us to eat. First, and most important to our survival, is the signal from our metabolic system telling us we are running out of energy reserves. That craving is real hunger we feel after at least a day of fasting. When we experience that craving, the high caloric value of the meal is not the objective; it's to replenish the calorie reserve. The higher the intensity of that craving, the less we care about how caloric or otherwise tasty the meal is. There is a wide range of intensity of that craving. Mild hunger is a gentle reminder that our body needs nourishment and manifests as a thought that pops up sometimes when our mind wanders. However, when we are busy, mild hunger typically remains hidden from our consciousness. At its peak intensity, however, the craving is almost constant and so intense that we will eat pretty much anything that we could identify as food. That craving is what we mean when we use the word hunger without qualifiers.

The second is the craving for extra energy. It encourages us to go over our calorie limit. That craving appears when we can acquire a high-calorie meal. Imagine a situation where you are not thinking about food, but then you are confronted with a highly-caloric meal. You don't even have to see it or smell it. You just need to know that it's available. Like that ice-cream you know that you have in your freezer or the peanut butter in the cupboard. When you see it or smell it, the appearance of that extra-calorie craving is almost instantaneous. Think walking into a doughnut shop or a fast food place. That craving also works its magic when we are already eating and know that we should stop, but we can't. That craving is at work when you reach for that extra slice of pizza or you can't stop eating your ice cream until you reach the bottom of its container. Let's call this craving binge hunger.

The third craving is for a specific nutrient. It's similar to the binge hunger but, obviously, it's aim is not calories. It's vitamins, minerals and other noncaloric nutrients that our body is lacking. That craving appears as a compulsion to add extra salt to your meal or when you unexpectedly choose a salad instead of your typical higher-calorie meal. Let's call this craving nutrient hunger.

The fourth kind of hunger is one that used to be practically unknown to our Stone Age ancestors. It manifests in us modern humans because we are trained to eat regular meals. Since we are used to the feeling of a full stomach, the sensation of an empty stomach makes us uncomfortable. Another factor of that hunger is related to our blood glucose and insulin fluctuations when we eat carbohydrate-rich meals. Ideally, your body's hormones, insulin and glucagon, keep your blood sugar at an optimal, steady level. However, because of our carbohydrate-rich diet, over time this regulation in many people becomes less than perfect. That results in an excessive fluctuation of our blood glucose level. Since glucose fuels the brain, we are sensitive to those fluctuations. When we feel that glucose level goes down and coincides with the feeling of an emptying stomach, we believe that we are getting hungry. That is the main reason we reach for snacks between meals. We also like those snacks to contain quickly-absorbing carbohydrates to steady our blood sugar level. We will call this craving false hunger.

The first three types of hunger were necessary for our ancestors' survival in the wild. The first one—true hunger or just hunger used to be most common for our nomadic forbears. It urged them to procure and consume their meals with different intensity depending on the exhaustion level of their energy reserve. If the intensity of the hunger wasn't high enough and the risk or difficulty of acquiring food was significant, our roving forefathers would just skip the meal altogether. Notice how our behavior differs due to our dependence on regular meals.

Nutrient hunger obviously helps guide us in food selection. If we are running out of vitamin c, for example, we would suddenly crave more onion. Our tastes for sourness and umami could help to guide us towards the foods that contain a particular nutrient profile.

The binge hunger used to be very important to our nomadic ancestors' survival in the wild. We have it because our roving forbears didn't have steady food supplies. The reason for binging is the instinct to store extra energy, and the result of the binge is us gaining weight. Notice that it's pretty common in mammals. For example, to survive the winter, the bear must build an adequate fat reserve to survive the period of hibernation when she doesn't eat. Our nomadic forefathers were, similarly to the rest of the animal kingdom, subject to the unpredictable nature of food availability. Sometimes they had more food than they could eat and sometimes not enough. Since they had to move from place to place, they couldn't carry with them sufficiently large food reserves. Another aspect of this problem was the difficulty of the preservation of extra food for storage.

The evolution "solved" these problems by using a method of storing their excess calories as body fat, which is common to other mammals. Having a reasonable layer of fat provided that critically important calorie buffer enabling them to survive periods without food. One could imagine, for example, Stone Age nomads gorging themselves with fruit and other carbohydrate-rich foods in the summer and fall before winter arrived. In the winter, due to the minimal availability of plant foods, unsuccessful or insufficient hunts meant undernourishment or starvation. That is when the stored layer of fat would become critically important. Without the gorging hunger, our species, even with all their extra mental power, could have gone extinct.

Obviously, binge hunger is the one which we could do without nowadays. With our steady food supply, we need not binge anymore like our ancestors did. However, we are still genetically nomads, and the binge hunger is part of the instinctual connection of our brains with metabolic systems. The instinct to overeat, due to its importance to survival, had to be strong enough to override the rationality of our ancestors. Now consider this: our nomadic forbears adapted their foods for consumption. However, how sweet was their fruit compared to ours? How refined were their starchy and fatty plants? How much salt did they have at their disposal to add to their meals? Did they have many seasonings? They probably processed their foods significantly by removing extra fiber, concentrate starches, fats, and sugars to make them tastier. Also, they could have added herbs to spice it up. However, the resulting taste enhancement couldn't have resulted in meals as enticing to our palate as our current calorie bombs. Imagine now that our craving is as intense as theirs, but our modern foods are much more binge-inviting. We have the same brains attuned to overeat moderately sweet, salty, starchy, fatty meals and we tempt them with those flavors cranked all the way up.

False hunger is obviously very destructive. It works mostly on people who already have problems with blood sugar regulation. These people are usually already overweight. Now, besides overeating their regular meals, they are constantly "hungry" between meals.

After we classified various kinds of hunger, let's see how they affect our everyday eating behaviors. Do we ever experience unqualified hunger? Most of us don't. Some of us have probably felt it fleetingly in its mildest form, but for the most part, we don't know that feeling. I, for one, didn't. As far back as I can remember, I always thought I was hungry in the morning. Nobody is unless they fast a day before. But, when we eat normally, we have a special metabolic reserve in our muscles and liver called glycogen sufficient for the best part of the day. However, the appetite for breakfast when it's sitting in front of you is genuine, but that craving is not hunger. It only arises when we put ourselves in a position in which high-calorie food is available and our stomach is empty. It's clearly a binge hunger. Do you know why I am so sure about it? There are no salads or other less energy dense meals on the morning menu. We are not hungry when we wake up. If we were, the salad would be as enticing to us any other meal. What do we like in the morning? Super caloric foods like eggs, bacon, buttered toasts, pancakes with syrup, orange juice, etc.

Although we can eat less caloric meals for lunch and dinner, that doesn't mean we are hungry. It's most likely nutrient hunger that makes us choose that salad over the burger once in a while. Obviously, it all depends on individual sensitivity to different types of hunger. Children, for example, are so motivated to resupply calories for their fast-growing bodies that their nutrient hunger manifests rarely. The underlying problem is that kids, like us, eat their meals on a schedule before they would naturally become hungry.

Our currently recommended regimen is not a natural one. Nobody claims it is. You can do a little research to confirm that. When you search for the natural diet or nutrition, you will find articles speculating what it could be. Even not precisely knowing what our natural diet is, we can say that our traditional regimen differs significantly from our natural one. Here is why. The default state for our nomadic forefathers was lack of food. For us, food is almost always within reach. For our roving ancestors, hunger was a motivator to obtain food and an encourager to eat it. We preemptively squash that feeling with breakfast and prevent its manifestation with our scheduled meals and snacks.

Here are some interesting questions: How do you think our nomadic ancestors felt while functioning during the day on an empty stomach? Were they miserable? Did they feel weak? Did they have a headache? Were they distracted by hunger?

The answer to all the above questions is no. Otherwise, you would have to admit that our ancestors, the farmers, corrected a huge evolutionary blunder by switching from our natural nomadic diet. If we assume that the natural state on the nomadic diet was an empty stomach, why do we feel uncomfortable in that state? I, for one, had always felt miserable when delaying my meals. I felt not only weak and uneasy but also usually developed a pounding headache when missing my feeding window. It seems like we are physically attuned to our three daily meals routine. Eating on a schedule feels just right.

You've heard about the nature vs. nurture debate. Nature refers to how we are genetically shaped. Nurture encompasses what we learn and how we adjust to our environment. Our eating behavior, like any other, is a combination of our genetics and the way we've learned to behave. Our parents trained us to eat regular meals. That training goes against our genetic adaptation. The amazing thing is how well we adjust to that unnatural eating schedule. Since we start that training from an early age, our brains grow accustomed to the feeling of a full stomach and all-day digestion. Conversely, we feel out of sorts to a different degree when our stomachs become empty.

We think that we are getting hungry. Our brains are very malleable at an early age, and, although we rebel, we get used to the scheduled meals. It becomes second nature to us. It feels so natural it never crosses our minds that it's a trained behavior. However, think about the consequences of that switch. The obvious ones are our heavy dependence on regular meals. That makes limiting calorie intake super hard which frequently leads to obesity. Then direct health implications affect even those of us who can stay within their optimal body weight limit. That is because the diet that we've been trained to follow is not optimal to our species.

Even though our brains can get used to the constant ingestions, our organs can't change their optimal operating mode. The mouth, esophagus, stomach, intestines, liver, gall bladder and pancreas work differently. They work extra hard to accommodate extra meals. The optimal timing to perform digestive functions also changes. Our metabolism and hormonal system, too, work unnaturally. I address the full implications of switching our eating framework in the later chapters.

CHAPTER FIVE

Menu Fluidity

Like many of us, I started paying attention to what I was eating when I got to a point at which I couldn't lose a few extra pounds and some bothersome minor health issues. That started for me a few years of experimentation and research to find the right mix of compounds or a diet that could help me. I went on a low carbohydrate diet, keto diet and fasted for different durations. I also tried different vitamins, minerals, amino acids, and other various compounds. Being a thorough experimenter, I also used many super foods.

In my enthusiasm to zero-in on the perfect supplement combo, I gathered so many compounds and potions I had to sequester a quarter of the refrigerator and a whole kitchen cabinet. However, I am not the one to settle for half measures. I was going all in. I didn't get discouraged after my initial setbacks. Instead of abandoning my experimentation, I broadened my search. To discover what to look for, I would watch videos of some well-informed MDs or chiropractors to discover what else I should try. That second phase of my research expanded my dispensary even further. As I was running out of space in the kitchen, I had to move my powders and pills to the large cupboard in the basement and used an extra refrigerator to expand my cold storage capacity. All this supplementation made sense to me. Smart people like Ray Kurzweil were doing precisely the same thing. Although I didn't get close to the impressive Ray's hundred pills a day, I did ingest a significant amount of powders, potions and pills. The methodology of adding potentially missing or otherwise beneficial nutrients made perfect sense. Even my not feeling a significant change in the way I felt wasn't bothering me too much. I believed that, in time, I would see the results. However, as a few months went by, I had my doubts. When I compared my experiences with the exalted praises I'd heard from the alleged experts; I just had to admit that none of the supplements worked for me.

Besides the supplements, I also experimented with diets. I felt noticeably better on the low carbohydrate and keto regimens when I switched from the standard carb-rich meals. Also, I tried fasting for different durations. That experience surprised me. Already at the end of the first day of fasting, my digestion worked differently. I felt physically better while fasting, except for the occasional headache. However, my mind couldn't shake the feeling I am depriving myself of my regular meals. Also, the sense of the empty stomach felt strange and triggered the thoughts about the missing meals. The most remarkable, however, was the discovery I don't feel hunger in the morning. I noticed the difference between thinking about food and being actually hungry.

Just about the time of my dietary experimentation, I pondered what would be theoretically the best diet for me, and a corollary to that—why do we have so many diets? My train of thought was as follows. After nearly ten thousand years of settled life, we couldn't have adapted to the steady grain-based diet which makes our pre-agrarian nomadic diet optimal for us. Therefore, of all the alternative regimens out there, the Paleo diet would make the most sense. However, after researching and trying that diet I realized that its effects weren't any better than other lower carbohydrate diets. I had a hard time staying within my calorie limit and gained weight on the Paleo diet. I couldn't stop munching on those tasty seeds and nuts. I was very disappointed that even eating similar foods to our nomadic forefathers didn't work for me. That realization seemed like a dead end on my quest for our optimal diet. I thought there is no single optimal diet, there are just nuances that suit certain people better than others. Therefore, all the dietary chaos out there makes sense. Everybody has to find their own marginally better diet and just live with it. I decided that the criterium regarding which way of eating is better is not an inherent capacity to make us feel better, rather to help us restrain overeating. Therefore, if _place the name of a diet here_ makes you eat less, that is your diet. However, I wasn't entirely satisfied with that conclusion. I still wanted to know how close we can get to emulating the nomadic diet of our predecessors today. Again, I was clinging to the conviction we are evolutionarily adapted to eat like them. Therefore, the nomadic diet is still our optimal diet. In that regard, the fact that our recommended regimen is based on carbohydrates clashed with my projection of the nomadic menu. They were not farming grains. Therefore, what are the chances it was their staple food? Virtually nil. Also unlikely was that they were finding enough tubers or other starchy plants to make their menu starch-based all year-round. Hence, their menu was definitely different than our modern menu. That line of thinking was bringing me back to the Paleo diet, which seems to be the closest to our pre-agrarian food choice.

After reflecting some more on our ancestors' survival in the wild, I realized that the accounts I had read about our ancestors' comfortable living couldn't have been representing their reality. When I was trying to imagine myself surviving in the woods without modern technology, I realized how smart our ancestors really were. Moving from place to place, roaming at different latitudes, able to survive ice ages, they had to make up for the simple technology they had at their disposal with their thinking. The fact that they survived in so many environments is amazing, but what and how they were eating was a big question. When I considered this, my first realization was that, even though the Paleo menu is probably in the ballpark of what they were eating, they couldn't have eaten it the way we do today. They couldn't have been choosing the composition of their daily meals. It was nearly impossible for them to have access to the same plant foods all year-round. The menu was changing from one place to another. It also differed with the seasons. Hence, eating according to the Paleo diet of nuts, fruit, meat, veggies, etc. in roughly the same proportions would be impossible for the real Paleolithic people. They would switch their foods wholly based on what they could find or hunt or fish. There would be periods of eating just meat or meat supplemented with veggies, only fruit, meat and nuts, and so on.

The variability of the menu throughout the year was a big factor in our nomadic nutrition. That obvious fact makes all our fixed macronutrient ratio diets suboptimal because our true nomadic menu was wildly changing in that regard. It would go from Keto to Paleo, to high carbohydrate. It would go from carnivorous, pescatarian and vegetarian. That fact explains why we can tolerate all those diets. Our roving forefathers lived on them, however, not all year-round on the same menu. The modern equivalent would be a few days of Keto, then a week or two low carbohydrates, followed by a few days with plenty of starches. The periods of staying on a particular macro-menu depended on where they were roaming. In warmer climates, there were probably more high carbohydrate periods, while in a colder climate, more low carbohydrate or keto.

Therefore, nowadays, whatever alternative diet we choose, it is only optimal for us for a while. After we stay on it too long, we are back in our modern, suboptimal mode. That fact also explains why many people feel better when switching diets. It doesn't matter from which diet to which, the change itself is what makes them feel better. Most people switch from the traditional high starch diet. Therefore, a low-carbohydrate, Paleo or Keto diet should work for them for a while.

One crucial aspect of our optimal diet is a radical variation of the macronutrient ratio. The specific foods should also vary as they did for our nomadic predecessors. When they changed their hunting and foraging areas, they would find different plants and different animals to harvest. I am not sure how relevant the fluidity of macro-ratios in our diet is to our health. However, a few implications immediately make sense. One is the health of our intestinal flora. Having limited high-carbohydrate periods and, most likely, more fiber than our current diet would make our GI tract microbes happy. Another one is our brain health. Usually glucose fuels our brains. For most of us on the standard carb-rich diet, it's the only brain fuel that our bodies use throughout our whole lives. However, our nomadic forebears would most likely go occasionally into ketosis whenever plant food was unavailable. Therefore entering that state sporadically may be optimal for the long-term optimal function of our brain.

CHAPTER SIX

Consumption Pattern

When I started convincing myself that our optimal diet should vary in its macronutrient ratios significantly, I was thrilled. Suddenly all the regimens we pursue and all their eventual ineffectiveness made sense. However, I discovered that it's not the only aspect of our ancestral diet that we've overlooked. There is something else that stands out when we try to picture the life of our nomadic ancestors. It's their eating frequency.

When considering the way nomads moved from place to place, mostly on foot, it's hard to imagine that they could carry a lot of things. They had to travel light. Yet, they had to bring some essentials; most likely the tools and weapons, maybe some skins to wear and for bedding. Bringing those necessities with them wouldn't leave much room for food. That realization is critical in our evaluation of their eating habits. They probably carried with them small quantities of dried or otherwise preserved food. However, that would be their emergency reserve. It would be their insurance policy if an unsuccessful hunt occurs or edible plants can't be found. Lacking significant enough food reserves used to compel our ancestors to prepare and eat food almost daily, and the necessity of obtaining and preparing food before consumption would make it impossible to eat frequently. The chain of activities comprising obtaining food, preparing it and then consumption had to be typical for our nomadic forbearers.

Therefore, eating on a frequent schedule is going against our natural eating pattern. Our ancestors would eat an extra caloric meal even when not hungry; but how often? Typically, they would have to gather or kill their future meal and then prepare it for consumption. Gathering wild vegetation, which wouldn't be as nutrient-dense as our fruit and veggies would require lots of walking, bending over and plucking. Hunting would be a similarly involved and even potentially risky activity. Preparing food for consumption wouldn't be effortless either. First, the nomads had to clean the harvested plants or animals and sometimes remove inedible parts. Then some mechanical processing was performed if necessary, like mashing, chopping and tenderizing. Then the meal would usually require cooking, which involved gathering woods, making fire and finally, cooking.

Yes, our roving forefathers were cooks, and they must have been quite skilled at preparing their meals. Remember the tools they had at their disposal and raw ingredients. We have a lot of cultivated plant food that is edible raw; they weren't so lucky. Most wild vegetation doesn't agree with our stomachs. Have you seen the comparison of wild bananas or wild carrots with their cultivated varieties? The difference is huge. We may consider our farmed veggies and fruits as processed by selective farming when compared with their wild counterparts. They had to prepare those plants themselves to make them digestible and nutritious enough. Most starches in tubers are hard to digest for us. That's why we cook our potatoes. Similarly, cooked grains suit us much better than raw. The same is true for us as it used to be for our pre-agrarian ancestors.

Remember, their teeth and stomachs weren't any sturdier than ours, but their caloric requirements were, because of that intensive work, most likely much higher than ours. They needed significant time to obtain and prepare food, and that process would have to be performed almost every day. Therefore, they would typically eat only one late meal, and that evening meal would be of variable caloric value. Depending on the quantity and quality of acquired foods, they would under-eat, overeat or go to bed hungry. When I first realized that nomads typically ate one meal I was surprised as I always assumed that our three meals daily is the requirement of our physiology. Hearing the mantra about the dangers of skipping meals sounds strange in that context. If we assume that one meal daily was optimal for our nomadic forefathers, it should still be optimal for us. I see that clearly when I put this in a different perspective. Our ancestors were active throughout the day, and when they had their meal ready in the evening, they would partake in the feast. By that time, they were quite hungry. It's not a coincidence we have a metabolic reserve in glycogen stored in our liver and muscles. Naturally, we should be using it during the day as our ancestor did.

Glycogen is basically glucose packaged for storage. Besides glucose, our body also stores fat as triglycerides and fatty acids. Our bodies are perfectly adapted to us functioning all day on those energy reserves. We can call this a form of a metabolic buffer. That buffer wasn't only used by our ancestors in an emergency. They used it every day. Our bodies are genetically adapted to use it. That is why we are not hungry in the morning. We start being truly hungry in the late afternoon as this reserve is depleted. Therefore, it makes sense we should listen to our body– obey the hunger signal instead of eating preemptively. We should work all day without interruptions and then eat to resupply our energy buffer.

What we do now is quite strange in comparison. We get up and eat breakfast, work for a few hours, then eat again, another few hours of work, then eat again. That frequent interruption of our routine for food breaks doesn't seem to make much sense. Add to that our coffee, soda, and snack breaks, and you'll see how our lives, in contrast to our ancestors', revolve around food. When I first compared those two patterns, my initial thought was that the reason must be the difference in the menu. Our nomadic ancestors were not relying on carbohydrates as their primary nutrient. Maybe that is the reason we eat piecemeal while consuming carbohydrates throughout the day. However, I discovered this is not the case. But, even when eating mostly carbohydrates, our body provides an energy buffering system in the mentioned glycogen. Conveniently enough, we store enough of that reserve fuel in muscles and liver to suffice for most of the day. So why need we eat breakfast in the morning while having this reserve? It is undoubtedly not physiologically necessary. If it is not required to eat breakfast and this is not the way we evolved to eat, why is it being recommended? Can it be just a tradition?

Please notice we are not famished in the morning. We are hungry when we have an appetite for a salad. Have you seen people eating salads in the morning? No, we eat the only meals we still crave when not hungry, the calorie-bomb—pancakes with syrup, eggs, bacon, bread, and butter, orange juice. By morning our stomachs are already empty, so there is no problem in wolfing down the big breakfast. However, should we? If we evolved not to eat breakfast, it means that our stomach should stay empty for most of the day. Our whole upper digestive tract should be at rest. However, health professionals tell us to pack it in in the morning. It's the most important meal of the day they say. It's the most harmful meal of the day.

Do you recall the adage: "Eat your breakfast alone, eat your lunch with your friend; give your dinner to your enemy." I think that they have it backward. I would give my breakfast to the enemy and have dinner for myself. The difference between skipping dinner and breakfast is very important. At first glance, one may think, *what is the difference? The period between the meals is still the same in both scenarios.* Here is the difference. We are not nocturnal animals. We are active during the day, and as our ancestors did, that is why we should function on an empty stomach. Again, here is my conjecture. A lot of hormonal activity is associated with digestion. Those hormones affect our brain. Therefore, we should rest and relax when we digest and be active on an empty stomach. That appears to be the way our pre-agrarian ancestors were operating and is also optimal for us.

Our feeding routine seems quite simple—we should eat when we are hungry. However, we modern people must remember that putting ourselves in the situation when an extra caloric meal is available will trigger the craving to acquire those extra calories. As with eating, it makes sense to assume that we should drink the same way, only when we are thirsty. Drinking that tea or coffee as a diversion or sipping absentmindedly from the water bottle just because it's within our reach is probably not a good idea. To check if it's optimal or not, we can think about our nomadic forebears again. How likely is it that, during the day, they would carry water containers just to stop and sip sometimes? Not likely. They were busy. They had things to do. They followed the thirst signal that reminded them when to drink. I can imagine that when they traveled, they would carry water reserves. However, as with the food ratios, water would be a precious commodity and dispensed only when necessary.

The unsteady availability of food and water was something that our nomadic forefathers had to adjust to. To mitigate that problem, they probably stayed close to water sources and carried some of it into unknown terrain. Similarly, they saved food surplus for emergency whenever possible. However, unlike settlers, they were limited on how much food and water they could carry with them. Therefore, occasionally, they had to endure periods of starvation and dehydration. Those involuntary breaks in eating and drinking used to be unavoidable. It makes sense that reasonably short periods of fasting and dehydration couldn't incapacitate our nomadic forefathers. Not eating for a few days or not drinking for a day or two shouldn't have a significant negative effect on their performance. Perhaps, up to a certain point, their mental, and physical performance, should be slightly better to increase their chances of survival. In that context, the reports of unusual mental clarity in the fasted state make perfect sense. Also, those occasional states of deprivation could be beneficial to our bodies as they allow many of our body's organs associated with digestive and urinary tracts extended rest and recuperation.

Our eating and drinking perspective as modern people is different as food and drink is almost always available. For some strange reason, we persuaded ourselves that putting extra food and water through our body is no big deal. It might or might not be. However, why not err on the side of caution? Why not use our bodies the way they've evolved to be used?

CHAPTER SEVEN

Misusing Our Body

What would happen if we used our digestive system closer to the way it evolved to be used? Maybe the frequency of the nutrition-related conditions like indigestion or constipation to severe like GI tract cancers would be not as high as it is now. Think about this: our digestive system apparently evolved to handle one big meal and, occasionally, rest entirely for a day or two. Now we fill it constantly all year-round. Due to the nature of consuming carbohydrates throughout the day, we rely, mostly, on metabolizing glucose that gets released quickly into our bloodstream after a carb-rich meal. That uneven supply of glucose and later insulin release occurs with every carb-rich meal and snack. That affects our brain. We use caffeine to steady out our alertness level. We drink coffee, tea and other caffeinated beverages for the wrong reasons. We need them because of our steady carbohydrate-rich diet that created that need. Have you noticed that we became practically dependent on coffee? All the reports about the beneficial properties of coffee seem a little suspicious. It's not a beverage which we evolved to consume. It may be slightly helpful on our unnatural diet; however, it may also disturb our natural rhythm of activity and relaxation.

Let's look at how our natural twenty-four-hour period should look. We should be able to become fully alert without the help of caffeine shortly after waking up, and we shouldn't be hungry. While abstaining from eating during the day, our body automatically supplies glucose to our bloodstream by steadily releasing glycogen from our muscles and liver. By late afternoon, we should deplete our energy reserve to the point of becoming hungry. Until then, the feeling of an empty stomach shouldn't bother us. Throughout the day we should be alert without the periods of sleepiness. When late in the afternoon we become hungry enough, we should be ready for an oversized dinner. We should be hungry enough to eat pretty much any meal. That is a great opportunity to have a healthy meal. After dinner, when your body releases all hormones related to digestion, you should become naturally relaxed, and within a few hours, after somewhat digesting your meal, you should become sleepy. During the night, your body will prepare an appropriate energy reserve to be available when you wake up. Depending on the fat, protein, and carbohydrate content of your dinner, you have either more glucose or fat-derived energy carriers waiting to supply you with energy throughout the day. Your body will match the needs of your muscles, brain and other organs with the available energy stored in your liver, bloodstream, and fat tissue. Your liver will produce extra glucose or ketones when needed.

Imagine your body, including the brain, and digestive and metabolic systems as a highly automated factory. Everything is tuned to an optimal way of operation. Your digestive system is optimized to being filled with one meal at the end of the day. The upper digestive system is optimized for resting during the day. Your brain functions at its best with the steady delivery of glucose or ketones from the body's energy buffering system, not directly from the carbohydrates shortly after ingestion assimilated and converted to glucose. Also, it is used to a certain hormonal cycle with the hormones relating to digestion working at rest. Can our body work in suboptimal conditions? Of course it can. However, the longer it operates in those less than optimal conditions, the higher the likelihood of something going wrong.

How does the constant, all year-round ingestion of carbohydrate-laden food affect our organs relating to digestion? Starting from our mouth where our saliva has problems neutralizing bacteria, feeding all the day on the steadily ingested carbohydrates, our whole GI tract is under attack by the not-so-friendly microbes. It's hard enough to keep our whole digestive tube in a microbial balance that is beneficial for digestion with one load of carb-heavy food. Now imagine the food keeps coming through our digestive system, and the starch or sugar is moistened by our saliva and warmed by our body. It's a microbial paradise. We have enzymes and our own beneficial microbes to fight the bad micro-invaders. However, look at the mouth as an example of how poorly our body can resist the microbial invasion. Even with daily brushing and flossing, we must go to the dentist periodically to remove the bacterial plaque. Also, as we get older, the periodontal disease frequently takes hold of our gums. There is also a whole range of conditions affecting our mouth, from abscesses to cancers. Between the intensified microbial activity and more frequent digestion, our whole GI tract is stressed more than it should be. Do you think that heartburn, for example, would be so common if we ate only once daily? How affected is our colon by not completely shutting down and being allowed to rest with an occasional full fast?

The body has limited resources. Yes, it can multitask. However, it is used to the periodic complete shutdown of our digestive tract. Our nomadic ancestors were fasting naturally many times a year. It was unavoidable. We don't. Imagine a factory not having maintenance breaks. Now imagine the factory being used above its original capacity. Keeping all the machinery running smoothly becomes difficult. Some machines, due to the constant use, perform poorly or even break down. That analogy, although simplistic, reflects well our misuse of our digestive system.

Let's go back to our body's need for maintenance.Notice that our body sometimes tells us explicitly to stop eating. This happens when we get sick. With an incoming fever, we not only lose our appetite but it's difficult to force us to eat. This is our body telling us, "I don't want to be bothered with digestion. I have to focus on fighting the disease," and what do our caretakers do? They make us eat, reasoning we need more energy to fight the disease. They don't consider that our body almost always has energy reserve. We can live for a few weeks without food. Therefore, a day or two without it can't harm us. However, distracting our body with digestion when it should give a hundred percent to fighting infection is definitely a bad idea.

Do you see the whole picture emerging of us working against our body? Starting from eating or drinking when we are not hungry or thirsty, through force-feeding ourselves when sick, we treat our body based on our simplistic understanding of what's good for us. We forget that our body is a super complex biological system, adapted over millions of years to work in an optimal way. Some of our adaptations are not specifically human. The one we sabotage with our regular ingestion is common in the animal kingdom. The availability of food varied for humans and for other animals. Sometimes there was too much, sometimes not enough. Therefore, occasional undereating, overeating and fasting is a natural part of living in the wild.

Here is another interesting point to consider—the issue of metabolic rate. I think that we got it wrong when we think that a high metabolic rate is an advantage. Metabolic rate is the amount of energy our body uses per unit of time. Let's say that we need a certain number of calories to perform a certain task. A higher metabolic rate means we need more calories than before to perform the same task. A high metabolic rate is considered good because it helps to lose weight. However, is it really good? Not necessarily, because the higher metabolic rate means that our body inefficiently uses food as an energy source. The higher the metabolic rate, the less efficient our metabolic system. As a consequence, our digestive system must process more food to produce the same energy.

We are being told that, when skipping meals, our metabolic rate decreases, which makes perfect sense because our body tries to be more efficient. If we still gain weight when eating fewer meals, the solution is not to eat extra meals but to eat less! From the evolutionary viewpoint, our metabolic rate should be as low as possible. Our nomadic bodies are optimized for efficiency. The "sloppiness" of our body when we eat extra meals may mean that our body is operating outside of its optimal mode. We like eating our meals, but our bodies didn't evolve to accommodate our eating pleasure. They are optimized for survival. This is the reason we gain weight. The extra nutrients are stored instead of being metabolized. If we crank our metabolism all the way up and exercise a lot, we can definitely lose weight quicker. However, how wise is it? According to some theories of aging, our metabolism contributes to aging. It is the oxidative damage during cellular metabolism. Therefore, eating more and exercising more than necessary is a good way to age faster and shorten our lives.

Even if we don't fully subscribe to this theory, we can look at our centenarians to see they eat moderately and are moderately active. They don't have big muscles and they don't run marathons. Their energy intake and expenditure is steady but moderate. That makes sense. We shouldn't abuse our digestion and metabolism. Yes, we can have huge muscles or jog all day while eating as much as we want and stay reasonably trim, but is it rational?

CHAPTER EIGHT

Training to Overeat

There are two aspects of our body's operation that make us think that we can tinker with its processes. First is its somewhat predictable behavior, and the second is its flexibility. Think about cigarette smoking. Compare the first reaction of our body to the tobacco smoke with how it feels to a longtime smoker. Isn't it astonishing that our body doesn't continue to react defensively to the toxic smoke? Why can the smoker inhale the noxious fumes all the way into his lungs without reflexive coughing? That is an example of a physical adaptation to adverse conditions. In the same way, as we know, our brain can adjust to adverse situations. Now imagine that we do something less traumatic to our bodies, like changing the timing of eating and drinking. Beyond the initial discomfort, our body will adjust to such a degree that the new schedule will feel natural.

Remember when you were a kid and your parents had to make you eat your meals? You were playing with your friends and then around noon, your mother would call you for lunch. While you were in the middle of your favorite pastime, you felt great. You didn't feel hunger. Your empty stomach not only didn't bother you, but you didn't notice it. Your brain wasn't telling you to stop. Your mother did. As kids, we naturally behave that way, and that is the time when that unnatural eating schedule bothers us. Some of us are more amenable to the consumption of regular meals than others. Those problematic kids—picky eaters—are more attuned to their bodies than most of us. They hate being forced to eat.

You see all those well-meaning parents worried about their kids resisting eating. We have gotten used to bizarre situations which we accept as normal. That mother sitting her infant child in a high chair and spoon feeding it. The porridge dripping from the kid's chin. The mother doesn't give up. She scoops it up and continues to put it in the child's mouth. When the child, frustrated, throws the food around, some of us find it funny. It isn't. A few years later, the child still resists. He still doesn't want to eat healthy, home-cooked meals. He won't eat broccoli and spinach. We misinterpret that behavior. The child instinctively won't eat low-calorie food when not hungry, however, he will eat French fries, a hamburger or a milkshake—

and for good reason; those are highly caloric meals and the child's instinct compels them to eat them just in case.

Parents use different tactics to make children eat. One of them is a pretend play. A parent makes airplanes from the food and tells a story about those planes needing to land in the best place, which is the child's mouth. Another one is bribery. The child would be able to watch more TV when he finishes his dinner. Yet another is a distraction. Mother plays the boy's favorite show on TV and, sneakily, when the kid is engrossed in the show, his mother forces the food into his mouth. Think about all those scenes of forced eating training which we consider normal. The resistance of children to frequent feeding is common. It is very rare for a child to enthusiastically eat regular meals. The children are behaving normally. They are genetically adapted to eat only when they are hungry. They would be just fine when fed only once daily. The hunger would make them eat, and the feeling of satiety would make them stop.

Looking at the feeding training logically, one must notice that we are making our kids into eating machines. How does that affect the kid's health? With all the developmental diseases that painfully affect our children, and we can't figure out a reason for the occurrence of, maybe, just maybe our unnatural eating pattern has something to do with that. For most of us, after a few decades of eating three meals daily, the switch to our natural food consumption pattern is not effortless. It becomes quite hard. The reason is our conditioning from early childhood to preemptive ingestion. After years of training, our eating schedule becomes second nature. Because the state in which we function throughout waking hours is associated with digestion, we accept that state as natural. In contrast to the way we behave when we are kids, an empty stomach, instead of comforting, makes us nervous. We develop strong negative associations with the feeling of an empty stomach. This is like any other adaptation to an adverse condition. It's no wonder that we can adapt to the unnatural eating pattern. Our brains can adjust to much more extreme situations.

We know about battered woman syndrome or Stockholm syndrome, when our brain adjusts itself to most bizarre situations. Although not as extreme as the adaptations mentioned above, our frequent eating adaptation is based on the same principle. After a sufficiently long conditioning, our full stomach all day long just feels right.

CHAPTER NINE

Listen to Your Body

Here is why we should refrain from eating and drinking ahead of feeling hunger and thirst. The human body is a dynamic biological system that regulates itself continually. It is very complex, and its internal processes are mostly unreadable to our conscious mind. Digestion is such a process, and it is one of many. Among others are activities related to removing the toxins and cellular waste. There are also operations associated with temperature control, immunity, and healing. The broadly understood healing is essentially maintenance – repairing or replacing damaged or underperforming cells. All those activities are coordinated and performed without our awareness and with varying intensity. Thus, our body reacts differently to a paper cut than to a deep wound. Depending on the severity of the damage, our body will deploy proper resources to remedy the problem. Consequently, some biological functions may gain priority, and some may lose it. The previously discussed loss of appetite when we come down with fever is the result of the nourishment resupply losing its prominence on the body's priority list.

Similarly to making us lose appetite, our body tries to influence other behaviors when needed. Notice another common request directed at our consciousness when we get sick. It is the directive to rest. Frequently, when we get sick, we feel not only weak but also drowsy. No matter the time of day,. when our body tells us to, we are able to sleep for long periods. Our body suppresses our natural circadian rhythm to allow that extra-long rest. Naturally, the details of the body's internal activities are not very transparent to us. Our consciousness is not bombarded continuously with the details of what's going on with our digestive, metabolic, or immune systems. We get only specific signals like pain, hunger, thirst, sleepiness or alertness when the body wants us to behave in a specific way; the same applies to the urgency of those requests. The intensity of the request signal is proportional to the gravity of the situation. Also, the absence of it is meaningful. When we are not commanded expressly to do something, it means that we shouldn't do it; that doing it spontaneously may not be optimal for us.

As humans, we can preempt our body's requests to provide food and water. Other animals can't do that because they are unable to reflect on their physiological needs. Therefore, they reflexively follow their bodies' prompts. We can anticipate some of our body's needs and attempt to satisfy them ahead of time. Let me give you an example. A dog drinks when thirsty. After getting an appropriately strong thirst signal, he promptly satisfies it. However, many of us drink our beverages all day long out of a habit, rather than when prompted by thirst.

We think that instead of waiting for a signal from the body, we should provide whatever we think the body needs ahead of time. And a satisfying way to do it is to drink regularly during the day. During the Stone Age, our ancestors couldn't drink regularly throughout the day because they didn't have water always within their reach. Consequently, they had to act the same way all other animals did – follow the body thirst and hunger prompts. But now we can sip that coffee, tea or water all day long. We don't only think that it's better for us to drink ahead of time, many of us consider the appearance of thirst as possibly harmful. Let's look at this from the body's perspective. If our body doesn't tell us to drink, it means that water stocks in the body are adequate. No extra water is needed. How does our body react when we have a drink at that time? It detects the extra water and promptly gets rid of the excess liquid by making us pee. We bother our digestive system and urinary tract for nothing. And, that is the best-case scenario. We don't consider the full extent to which we could sabotage our body's normal operation by preemptive drinking. It is possible that we deprive our urinary tract of the resting period which could be used for healing or fighting infections. Of course, our body gets rid of extra water and works around our drinking schedule to perform its other functions. But how optimal is it?

It's strange how differently we perceive our body's prompts when it comes to bathroom visits. We consider it unhealthy to hold it or force ourselves to go beforehand. We believe it is best when we do it as soon as we get the signal to go. We don't see that the hunger and thirst signals constitute another side of the same coin. We should obey all calls concerning physiological functions ASAP. However, while going to the bathroom was possible on very short notice for our nomadic ancestors, obeying thirst and hunger signals wasn't always immediately achievable. Namely, food and drink weren't always at hand. Therefore, some time was needed to acquire them. Because of that, there has to be a natural safety margin associated with obeying those signals. We don't absolutely have to eat or drink immediately after becoming hungry or thirsty. We can supply our body with food and drink during a certain reasonable period without harming ourselves. That is a significant point. We should not interpret moderate hunger or thirst as an urgent warning. Instead, we should see it as a cue that our body is ready to accept food and water; the important word here is *ready*.

Let us illustrate how potentially harmful our preemptive eating and drinking is. Picture a procedure that involves loading something on one conveyer belt and unloading from the other. In between, an operation takes place. The operation is quite involved and takes a significant amount of time. That is a simplified view of the digestion process. When we supply a meal to our digestive system, we start a complex operation. Imagine how important timing is to the thorough processing of the meal moving along our GI tract. First, the meal must spend enough time in our mouths, to be sufficiently moistened and chewed. Then it must spend an appropriate amount of time in the stomach to be churned and broken down chemically. Subsequently, after getting more enzymatic treatment from the liver, it continues its journey through the intestines. All these require accurate timing during each stage of the process.

There is a reason why extracting nutrients happens at a relatively slow pace. Those nutrients once obtained from the preprocessed food have to be distributed to appropriate organs in our body. Consequently, one element of the processing chain relies on the next one. It seems reasonable that second-guessing that multi-stage complex operation is not advisable. It's best to rely on the body's own control of the digestive process. In short, beyond waiting for the signals of hunger, thirst, and when we have to go to the bathroom, we shouldn't be concerned with the exact timing of the digestion process. And, we should interpret properly the signals of hunger and thirst. Hunger means that our GI tract is ready to receive nourishment. To be exact, it means that the digestive operation is at the stage at which extra food can be accommodated.

Let's be specific. We are talking here about the signal of unqualified hunger. That feeling signals to our consciousness the full readiness of the GI tract. Note that the binge hunger will kick-in regardless of the digestion stage of our previous meal, as it arises in our brain based on the perceived attractiveness of the potential meal. Of course, the binge hunger is stronger when it coincides with our empty stomach; like in the morning when it's time for breakfast. What does it mean when we eat breakfast before receiving the proper hunger signal? It means that our body is "willing" to compromise to a certain degree the digestion of yesterday's dinner to acquire the precious extra calories from breakfast. Please note that when eating additional meals, our metabolic rate rises, which means that we are not getting maximum calories from that extra meal.

Pondering this behavior, we can see how well our bodies are adapted to the uneven availability of food; we can fast and also be encouraged to overeat and tolerate reasonably well occasional overeating. That means that we can accommodate a sufficiently attractive meal in the middle of our digestion cycle. Our digestion won't be optimal, but we will acquire extra energy. That is a great survival strategy. However, the additional meal consumption which used to be an exception for our nomadic forefathers became the norm for us modern people. Nowadays, this behavior is routine, and to be able to function with the unnaturally full belly, we need to train ourselves to feel reasonably comfortable accompanied by steady digestion. However, that spurious comfort while eating frequent meals is deceiving. It's much better to fully cooperate with our digestive system instead of somewhat undermining it with continual eating and drinking. As our nomadic ancestors did, we should trust our body's signaling to tell us when to resupply it with food and water.

In the case of our preemptive eating, as previously mentioned, we technically eat when we are hungry. However, instead of waiting for real hunger, we stage the appearance of a different craving. We invite the binge hunger by putting that sumptuous meal on the table, or by visiting a restaurant. We use our extra calorie acquisition instinct, to make ourselves eat additional meals. And the timing of those additions when it comes to breakfast and lunch is unfortunate, because as mentioned before, our digestive system is not entirely ready to accommodate extra food. As per our nomadic adaptation, our upper GI tract should be resting during most of the day.

Coming back to the various intensities of hunger, we may look at it this way: If we are just slightly hungry at the end of the day, it means that our body is involved in a more important activity; that there is a valid reason for pushing ingestion to the background.

Whatever our body is preoccupied with, it makes sense to skip the meal to let it focus on the problem. In that context, we can regard our level of hunger as a crude indicator of our health status. That very thought may have motivated someone to coin the phrase healthy appetite. Thus, your hearty appetite at the end of the day means that replenishing your energy reserve is the first priority for your body. And, that is a good thing. Unfortunately, we won't be able to see the nuances of hunger if we suppress it with eating regular meals. We ought to stop trying to outsmart our body with simplistic "improvements". It is arrogant of us to think that we can second-guess the super-complex biological system we call the human body by feeding it on our terms. Instead, we ought to confidently follow its cues. We should start listening to our bodies again.

CHAPTER TEN

The Salad Test

When we should eat? Obviously when we are hungry. However, as explained in previous chapters, the feeling of different cravings can be confusing. Especially when trained to eat on schedule. To determine if we are really hungry, we can perform a simple mental exercise that will give us the answer. Mind you, you can perform it with any low-calorie meal, I, however, use a bowl full of lettuce. I call it the salad test.

Here is the theory behind the Salad Test. Genuine hunger appears only when we crave low-calorie meals. Therefore, anytime we think that we should eat, we can verify it by thinking about substituting the meal we crave for a less caloric meal. If we still are in the mood to eat the less enticing substitute, we are genuinely hungry. Unless you are addicted to lettuce, picturing a salad without dressing and comprised of mostly lettuce should work well. If you are an eager lettuce eater, you may substitute it with your own least favorite low-calorie food. It is critical to perform the test before starting to eat because when we start eating a highly nutritious or caloric meal, it's usually too late to stop. The craving for dense calorie carriers is super strong.

Based on the salad test, it's easy to skip breakfast. The only problem when skipping a meal is the feeling of deprivation. That feeling is related to our three-meal training. It's the combination of the strange feeling of an empty stomach and thoughts that we are missing something that is important. When I was going through that phase of switching to the natural diet, I was genuinely feeling sorry for myself. My brain was playing tricks on me. In my mind, I felt so close to being hungry that I was ready to give up. The smell and view of a sumptuous breakfast combined with the feeling of the empty stomach were overpowering. In my case, I don't remember how often I broke down and ate a token breakfast, but I am sure there were a few. For me, that feeling of deprivation combined with thinking about my empty stomach as something unnatural lasted for a month or two. It was the strongest—requiring significant willpower—for the first week or two. After a few months of eating dinner only, the feeling of deprivation diminished to where I could watch a person eating eggs, bacon and buttered bread in the morning and feel almost neutral. It's a strange feeling getting to the point that the empty stomach not only doesn't make you uncomfortable but gives you a peaceful feeling.

Now when I reflect on it, that feeling makes perfect sense. Over time, that comfort with an empty stomach stretched for me to where, when I was busy, I would occasionally forget about dinner, and then, at about seven or eight, it's easy to skip dinner altogether.

I used the salad test initially when switching to the natural diet. After a while, however, I didn't have to use that imaginary bowl of lettuce. At a certain point, calorie bombs stopped having the same effect on me. As with frequent feeding adaptation, it was possible for me to adapt back to the natural eating-when-hungry schedule within a few months. Not thinking about food during the day is great as one can fully focus on daily tasks. Also, the extra time not spent on preparing and consuming the extra meals is a bonus. Now you may stay in bed longer or use that extra time in the morning for a brisk walk. The lunch break is also nothing to sneeze at. It can be used for walking or running errands. When skipping breakfast and dinner, in addition to gaining some time, you'll also be eating less food, which means that you can focus more on the quality of your meal. Also, obviously you'll have less cleanup. Your kitchen chores will be amazingly easy to perform. If you decide on a one course dinner, you'll have only one plate to wash. Obviously, you can continue cooking fancy meals if that's your thing. However, since I switched to the natural diet, I noticed that my taste has changed. I am much more satisfied with simple meals. Every time I eat my dinner, it tastes great.

There are other aspects of the natural eating model that I find interesting. One of them is the short window in which I think about food. Even when eating carbohydrates, I don't feel the pronounced cravings for seconds. Also, as much as I enjoy the process of eating, after the last bite, the thoughts of food disappear from my mind. Also interesting is how quickly I wake up in the morning. The grogginess that I always experienced when getting up is gone and so is my continually stuffy nose.

And then there is the clear distinction between the way my body and mind feel before and after the meal. The dinner becomes a dividing line between alertness and relaxation. When we function eating three meals daily, we blur this natural dividing line, and as a result, we become less alert when working and less relaxed when we rest. This muddling of our natural state may be also responsible for our frequent sleeping problems.

CHAPTER ELEVEN

Eating Tactics

For me, switching to the natural way of eating was relatively painless. It was mostly a mental challenge. I hardly felt hunger, and the empty stomach didn't bother me. However, I was a little distressed with the thought I was missing my meals. From my perspective today, thinking about deprivation in the context of missing breakfast seems bizarre. Yet, at the time, it felt real. I remember vividly grieving for my first meal of the day. I imagined myself eating a sumptuous breakfast, and as I did that, I was thinking, *I could be having this delicious meal but instead, I am sitting here not eating.*

That knowledge of missing a deserved pleasure used to trigger many longing thoughts about food during the day. I could tell I was physically okay, even better than okay. My empty stomach felt much better than typically after a meal. Yet, thoughts of eating popped up during the day. That divergence of the physical feeling of wellbeing and uncomfortable thoughts of missed eating opportunities was strange. Now as I fast during the day, I notice how nuanced the feeling of hunger is. Typically, until around two o'clock, I don't have thoughts about food at all. After that, the ideas about eating pop up sometimes; however, they are not too intrusive. Starting at around four, they become stronger, but still, their intensity varies. Sometimes they are more apparent, and sometimes even barely noticeable. There are days that my hunger is barely strong enough to motivate me to eat. When those days coincide with my particularly busy schedule, they create a perfect opportunity for all day fasting.

Here is one aspect of our ancestors' behavior I grasped only when I understood what independence from regular meals really means. Although obtaining food was vitally important for our ancestors, the eating itself wasn't their obsession, it was just another physiological activity that had to be satisfied. They weren't chained to steady eating the way we are. Being satiated meant that the next meal was just an option, like any other. They could clearheadedly decide against eating if obtaining food was too risky or there were other more pressing matters like finding shelter. Contrast that behavior with the exigencies of our modern lives. We are practically chained to our meals. I can't count the times where I had to sit at a dining table when I wasn't hungry.

As they say, appetite comes with eating, and it does. It is much easier to abstain from eating completely than to start eating and stop. However, in social situations, we are compelled to eat. Our culture exerts enormous pressure on us. From everyday meals at home when we sit to breakfast, lunch, and dinner together as a family, to a company meeting where pizza is served, there is a pressure to participate in communal meals. Perhaps our nomadic forebears were undergoing the same pressures. Yes, they were most likely also eating together. However, because of their circumstances, they were doing it much less frequently. They would share dinner as a group, but all participants were sufficiently hungry. Imagine that our bodies adjusted themselves to that natural sparser, hunger-driven, eating cycle for millions of years.

After a while of routinely skipping breakfast and lunch, eating just dinner feels natural. However, unlearning scheduled eating may be difficult for some people. After decades of eating almost constantly all day, getting used to having your belly empty can be a challenge, but after a few months of eating just dinners, your mentality will change. You will understand what it means to be free from the constant thinking about food, and you'll see how accurate is the nature-intended fueling of our brains and muscles. Steady is the word. Your body's natural energy buffer will dose glucose precisely to your brain and muscles, and when you reduce your carbohydrate consumption, your body will produce required fuels from other macronutrients. Also, you will see how easy it is to change your menu and reduce your calorie intake. When you are finally ready for dinner, you'll be hungry, exactly as you should. And you won't have to put loads of condiments or seasonings on your food to improve its taste. This is interesting—adding extra flavorings won't be as enticing as it used to be when you were eating three meals daily. Back then, you needed extra incentive to eat all your meals—adding ketchup or salad dressing worked great for that purpose. Now, you'll appreciate the taste of your meal's basic ingredients. You will be surprised how good plain lettuce tastes.

Because you'll eat various meals with similar enthusiasm, limiting calorie intake and switching proportions of fat, carbohydrates, and protein in our meal will become much easier than on the traditional diet. There is an ideal diet and then there is real life. The natural human diet is irregular. It is fluid in the ratios of fat, protein, and carbohydrate content. It is also variable in food selection and daily caloric intake. Although our nomadic forefathers ate usually one meal a day, there were days when they ate more frequently, and those days when they fasted. Our bodies are made for the variability of our sustenance. Therefore, we shouldn't panic when we occasionally vary our eating schedule.

We should realize the hierarchy of the importance of our dietary behaviors. One meal daily is somewhere near the top of the list. The second place, which makes it important, is making dinner that one meal. Then there is variability of macronutrient ratios—changing our meal's profile from carb-rich to fatty. Especially important is to occasionally go into ketosis. Unlike with a low-carbohydrate diet, the high carbohydrate regimen feels very normal to us. The starchy menu is the one we naturally gravitate toward. Our bodies crave carbohydrates because it's a quick-absorbing and quick-metabolizing nutrient. Our brains love carbohydrates as they provide a rapid glucose supply to our energy-craving cerebrum. Powerful cravings for carbohydrates and especially sugars made perfect sense for our nomadic ancestors. However, that doesn't mean they should be our main macronutrient all year-round. Therefore, we should remember that meals containing concentrated carbohydrates are a perfect inducement for overeating.

We can imagine that surviving winters for nomadic humans was a challenge. Between the increased caloric needs due to the colder weather and inability to fall back on plant food, it wasn't easy to survive the colder months of the year. Since they couldn't have carried with them food stocks, their strategy would be similar to other mammals faced with that problem. Notably, they would store their energy reserve as body fat. Yes, carrying a reasonable layer of fat for a few months seems natural. The perfect term for that strategy is "scheduled obesity." Our nomadic predecessors would overeat at the end of summer and fall to enter winter with a few extra pounds. Those few extra pounds were their insurance policy for surviving the winter. That is where the carbohydrates would play their role. The end of summer and fall would provide an excellent opportunity to graze on fruits, nuts, tubers, and other carb-rich plant foods. Our ancestors would be hooked on those carbohydrates. They couldn't get enough of them. However, this addiction had to end with the end of the availability of carbohydrate-rich foods. Therefore, perhaps we evolved to overeat on carbohydrate-rich foods to such a degree we gain weight. It also makes sense we haven't developed natural brakes to stop gorging on carbohydrate-rich foods. The seasonal change would do it for us. The carb-rich foods would disappear from our reach with the end of fall. Now, we grow our carb-rich foods all over the world. We have hothouses and silos full of fruit and grain. How coincidental is it we have carb-rich food all year-round and we overeat all year-round? The result of that programmed behavior was as predictable for our nomadic ancestors as it is for us. Our ancestors were probably slightly overweight throughout the winter, while most of us are overweight to a different degree all year-round.

From that relationship between the addictive nature of carbohydrates and obesity, we should draw conclusions regarding our dietary tactics. We should be very cautious about refined carbohydrates. Here is a little warning about the high carbohydrate diet—it's addictive. Similar to sugar, starches—especially combined with fats can cause cravings that last a few weeks. During that high carbohydrate sensitivity mode, it's difficult to eliminate starches and sugars from the menu. According to dieters attempting to switch from a high to a lower carbohydrate diet, the transition is difficult. Even after the change, while eating lower carbohydrate meals, we are still strongly attracted to carbs. It takes a few weeks until choosing non-starchy meals becomes easier.

Probably the best tactic would be to emulate the behavior of our nomadic forebears. Therefore, we should limit our carbohydrate-heavy dining to one a few months long. Throughout that period, we could overindulge as our ancestors did. We can do that, with our continuous availability of carbohydrates, any time throughout the year. However, it would make sense to do that, as our ancestors did, in the late summer and early fall. Although we could switch in and out of the carbohydrate-heavy mode weekly, it may not be a good idea. The difference between seasonal and weekly macronutrient switch is how often we have to fight the temptation of carbohydrate-rich foods.

To accomplish the seasonal menu changes, we could think of it as switches between various popular alternative regimens. Those seasonal diets would offer variable fat, protein and carbohydrate ratios as in the ketogenic, high carbohydrate and Paleo diets. Among them, the ketogenic diet seems of special importance to our long-term health as it was typical for our ancestors to stay on a similar high-fat regimen for one or more months of the year. This diet is unlike other diets in its effect on our brain because our cerebrum is not fueled with glucose but ketones while on it.

Throughout the rest of the year, we should follow a moderate carbohydrate diet similar to the Paleo diet. How perfect is that? Moderate carbohydrates provide enough glucose for the brain. Therefore, for about three quarters of the year, our brain is fueled by glucose with a short break for a keto brain reset. This wintery total break from carbohydrates could be very important for our mental health.

Think about eating as Stone Age humans did in this way. Eating behaviors were dictated by external circumstances and genetics. Our eating behaviors were shaped by our nomadic forebears' living circumstances. We inherited the genes, but our circumstances are completely different. For our roving ancestors, the change of diet was dictated by the availability of certain foods. We don't have that constraint anymore. We can get pretty much any food at any time. Therefore, we must force ourselves to do the switch. Lowering carbohydrates in our meals is such a conscious switch and it's a difficult one. To stay the course of the natural diet, a cheat is sometimes helpful. Ideally, when we get up in the morning, we should eat nothing. To start the transition, we can still keep drinking coffee in the morning. It's not much, however, a little cream in the coffee can ease the transition. It worked for me.

Let's talk about weight control while on our natural diet. One would think that while eating just one meal daily we would have trouble maintaining our weight. We would lose pounds quickly.

Unfortunately, that is not the case. The nutritionists are correct about the fact that when skipping meals our metabolism slows down. This is similar to the situation that all dieters face when they lower their food intake. Our metabolism compensates for the reduced inflow of calories by squeezing more energy from the same amount of food. Many nutritionists consider this a bad thing because it gets in a way of quickly losing weight. That reaction of the body makes perfect sense as the better efficiency (that is, a lower metabolic rate) should be the best course of action when faced with limiting food availability.

If lowering the metabolic rate doesn't otherwise compromise our body's functioning, it's the best course of action. The higher metabolic rate when we eat additional meals seems abnormal from the Stone Age nomadic perspective. Due to a lower metabolic rate, when eating one meal daily we need not make it the size of a combined breakfast, lunch and dinner. We can just have a somewhat oversized dinner in place of three meals worth of food. When we compare that to our traditional three meal eating plan, we can plainly see we not only eat too frequently but we eat also too much food, and that is not without its consequences. Our digestive system must process all that extra food that doesn't provide extra energy to our body. Think about what it means to our caloric requirements. On the natural diet, we must take into account our lower caloric expenditure and therefore reduce the portions of our dinner.

Let's return to losing weight. The natural regimen, although closer than any other diet, is not a miracle diet. That means we have to watch calories the same way as when on any other diet. However, keeping track of what you eat and how much you eat becomes, you guessed it—three times easier. In all seriousness, it's trivial to vary your foods and adjust portion sizes when following our natural regimen because you have only one meal to deal with. There are so many advantages to eating dinner only for adjusting calories and changing macronutrient ratios that nothing else even comes close. Think about this. You eat your meal at the end of the day. At that time, you know exactly what your level of activity was. If you were running a marathon, you pack it in. If you were sitting at home and reading a book, you just eat a medium salad.

You can go as fine-grained and scientific about your dieting as you want. You can weigh your food or buy a plate with rule markings on it to give you some idea about the volume of the food on your plate. You are in control. You can eat your dinner at home, and you can easily and precisely dose your calories. Eating at a restaurant is also easy as, nowadays, menus list the caloric value of meals.

Here is my experience with weight loss while following the natural regimen. Unlike on the traditional three meals daily diet, the weight loss is almost immediate. The reason is most likely that eating only one meal daily we are functioning at the lowest metabolic state. On the traditional diet, when we reduce our calorie intake, our metabolic rate goes down. On our natural diet, our metabolic rate is already low, therefore the weight drops quickly. For me, when I am not very active physically, reducing my dinner to the size of my pre-diet-switch dinner results in a reasonably fast weight loss.

Another important thing to note here is that, once you are adapted to one meal, you don't feel hunger in the same way. It's not as intrusive. Because you're comfortable with your empty stomach, the only manifestation of hunger is a very mild hint sometimes, and that hint comes when your attention is unoccupied. When you're busy you may easily forget about your meal. It makes perfect sense that the feeling of hunger manifests differently when functioning on a natural diet. It can't be too intrusive. If it were, it would interfere too much with the activity we are engaged in, and that activity, for the nomadic human could be directly related to acquiring food. Too strong of a hunger signal could sabotage the food acquisition effort.

From the perspective of a person following a traditional diet, it's hard to understand the freedom from the thoughts related to food that comes with switching to the natural diet. Think about it this way. Since we've evolved with the sporadic food supply, living with an empty stomach was a norm, the same way we feel with our stomachs full all the time. We already know how to determine if we are truly hungry—we can just do the salad test. Obviously, usually once a day in the late afternoon we can pass the test. When we do, it's time for dinner. This is when another advantage of the natural diet manifests itself—namely, we are hungry enough to eat a less caloric meal. Which is great because it means it is also not that difficult to switch the macronutrient ratio.

A sure-fire way to quickly drop a few pounds while eating only the dinner is to simply swap our usual highly caloric meal for a salad. One of the biggest advantages of eating dinner only is the reduced temptation to overeat as it happens only once daily. That combined with the mild manifestation of hunger and ease of keeping track of the ingested calories makes our natural diet perfect for controlling one's weight.

Let's sum up the framework of our natural diet.

The general rule is to eat when hungry and drink when thirsty. That advice should result in us eating one meal daily, drinking sparingly (if you are excessively thirsty, you may have a health problem) and occasionally fasting. We should vary our meals significantly in macronutrient ratios. We should move between high carbohydrate and low carbohydrate menus all the way to keto.

Conclusion

Let me recapitulate my simplified view of why it's important to follow our natural eating pattern. The reason is to give the digestive system time to properly digest the consumed meal. If we evolved to have one meal every twenty-four hours, it means that our upper digestive system should be at rest for most of the day. That has consequences for all organs related to digestion. From our mouth, esophagus, stomach, liver, gallbladder, pancreas and intestine, this once daily engagement is the optimal pattern of operation. Imagine these days our organs working three times more frequently than they should.

Now let's look at our metabolism.

We've evolved to be supplied with energy by our metabolic buffer. The carriers of that energy are stored fat or glycogen in our muscles and liver. Our body should be in charge of the timing and dosage of the metabolic fuels—glucose, ketones or other derivatives of fat. Our body "knows" best when and how much of those fuels we need. They will be distributed in exact amounts to our muscles, brains and other organs as needed.

Now contrast that operation with the one when we consume extra meals. In that scenario, the upper digestive system must engage every few hours to process the incoming foods. When the meal contains significant carbohydrates, those assimilate fast and can cause a rise in blood sugar level, which has to be counteracted with insulin. Our body's energy buffer must limit the dosage of glucose from the glycogen reserve due to the influx of extra glucose directly from the GI tract. The result is a significant interference with the natural operation of both our digestive and metabolic systems.

The disruptive effects of extra meals can be handled just fine by our body, at least for a few decades. After that, which means thousands of extra meals digested, both the digestive and metabolic autoregulation somewhat loses its effectiveness. After hitting forty or fifty, we feel the results of that deregulation. Our mouth can't keep up with the bacteria feeding on the constant flow of starches and periodontal disease begins. Our esophagus develops acid reflux disease from the constant flow of sustenance. Our stomachs fare no better. Ulcers and other problems develop. Because of the overworked pancreas, our blood sugar regulation suffers. Our liver is also compromised by trying to keep up with the incoming three-daily-meals. Our intestines are not having any rest and operating out of their optimal zone and develop many problems. Among others, they can't effectively resist the hostile microbes. That cripples our immune system. Our look changes as our skin shows signs of compromised metabolism and immunity.

We don’t know how much our unnatural diet affects our health and I am not aware of scientific studies comparing the effects of our natural diet to the current one. Therefore, somewhat simplistically, I have to evaluate the two based on logic and the way I feel and look. When I look at my face, I can't believe the difference in how my skin looks and feels as compared to how it looked a year ago. The same is true of the steadiness of my mood and alertness of my mind. Now I take for granted the steady feeling of wellbeing throughout the day. No pains and discomforts of any kind. However, unlike before I feel hunger. It shows up, as it should, in the late afternoon and makes me enjoy my dinner. After the meal, I feel naturally relaxed, and after a few hours, I feel sleepiness coming on. I am convinced that my current routine is the natural human eating pattern. Based on that, I can't escape the thoughts of the societal impact of our unnatural dietary training. How many physical and mental conditions that occur in our society can be related to our unnatural diet? How does the total exclusion of ketosis from our lives affect the development and continual operation of our brains? Is our susceptibility to addictions related to our unnatural diet? To what degree is our off-balance intestinal flora compromising our immunity? What effects has our suboptimal nutrition on our kids' development?

We have nomadic bodies attuned to the less frequent ingestion and more variable nutrient menu. After we domesticated ourselves, we ate more frequent meals that contain unvarying macronutrient proportions. That radically different model of food consumption based on early agrarians' idea of how they should consume their crops is now our nutritional foundation. We can forgive our ancestors for creating the practical, albeit flawed, concept of nutrition. They didn't realize the consequences of the change, and their goal was to feed more people predictably, but we live in the twenty-first century, and we shouldn't pretend we don't see the difference between natural and unnatural nutrition. Don't get me wrong. I think that everybody has a right to eat any way they like. However, the nutritional standard must change. We shouldn't support the food consumption model which relies on us being trained from infancy to change our natural eating behavior.

If you took away only one concept from this book, I'd like for it to be one image. The scene of a toddler throwing or spitting her food out in defiance of the frequent-eating training. You know, like the one you often see in commercials. This picture is neither cute nor funny. It's the symbol of our innate resistance against the unnatural diet forced on us from early childhood.

About the Author

"The people with ideas have no power
and the people with power have no ideas..."

—Harmon Okinyo

Gregory Stypko was born in Gdansk, Poland, and was privileged to witness firsthand the birth of the Solidarity movement in the city in 1980, led by Lech Wałęsa. During that period, Gregory was interned by the communist authorities as an untrustworthy citizen.

Following graduation from the Technical University of Gdansk with a degree in Hydro Acoustics, Gregory emigrated to the United States. There, he has worked as a hardware and software engineer for startups and established corporations in various engineering and managerial roles. He lives with his girlfriend and their dog near the Jersey Shore.

When he has time to himself, Gregory enjoys reading or listening to books; he is fascinated by quantum physics and astrophysics. He has an interest in history, with a particular curiosity about ancient Rome and the late 19th and early 20th centuries.

Gregory also loves sports, is learning to play the piano and is always trying to improve his knowledge of other languages, including French and German, in which he regularly gets his news.

Gregory has always appreciated “out-of-the-box” thinking and the power of ideas. He has written for a low-carb food blog in the past.

You can contact Gregory Stypko at gregstypko@gmail.com.

Made in United States
Troutdale, OR
11/03/2026

56847388R00056